THREAD LIFTS FOR BEGINNERS

Comprehensive Guide To Non-Surgical Facial Rejuvenation, Techniques, Benefits, And Aftercare Tips

DR SAWYER DIEGO

DISCLAMER

Nothing in this book should be interpreted as medical advice; it is meant exclusively for educational reasons. Regarding their specific health issues and treatment options, readers are urged to speak with licensed healthcare professionals. The publisher and author disclaim all liability for any errors or omissions in the material provided, as well as for any negative effects that may arise from using or abusing the information. Although every attempt has been taken to guarantee that the material in this book is correct as of the date of publishing, new research may have superseded some of the content because medical knowledge is always changing. It is recommended that readers confirm the most recent medical recommendations and guidelines. The reader of this book undertakes to release the author and publisher from any claims or liabilities resulting from the use of this information, and understands and accepts the inherent risks connected with healthcare decisions.

TABLE OF CONTENTS

ABOUT THE BOOK

With its ability to rejuvenate facial contours without the invasiveness of traditional surgeries, "Thread Lifts for Beginners" provides a thorough introduction to thread lifts for those who are considering this minimally invasive cosmetic procedure.

 The book starts by defining what a thread lift is, outlining its historical development, and contrasting it with other facial rejuvenation techniques like Botox and dermal fillers.

Preparation is one of the most important topics discussed because it is critical to achieving the best possible results. Readers are led through pre-procedure discussions with cosmetic surgeons, comprehending treatment plans, and making the necessary mental and physical preparations. Safety factors, such as possible risks and anticipated outcomes, are carefully described to assist people in making decisions.

The book includes information on anesthesia options, pain management strategies, and a detailed description of what to expect during the thread lift procedure on the day of the procedure. It also emphasizes immediate post-procedure care instructions so that readers are aware of how to handle swelling and initial discomfort and follow the required restrictions for the best possible recovery.

The recovery and aftercare section discusses long-term care strategies and how to maintain skin quality and facial contouring over time. It also offers advice on how to manage discomfort and post-procedure restrictions. Finally, it discusses the significance of follow-up appointments.

Additionally, "Thread Lifts for Beginners" explores the psychological effects of aesthetic enhancements and potential cost savings compared to more invasive surgical options, all of which are supported by patient success stories and satisfaction rates. It also highlights the many benefits of thread lifts, including their immediate and long-term effects on facial appearance and skin quality.

In addition, the book guides on selecting qualified providers, assessing clinic facilities, and comprehending pricing and payment options so that readers can make well-informed decisions. It also provides insights into managing and minimizing these risks as well as ethical considerations related to aesthetic procedures.

In addition, non-surgical face rejuvenation options are reviewed along with their advantages and disadvantages in comparison to thread lifts; lifestyle modifications for skin health and customized treatment regimens are also examined to help readers attain better aesthetic outcomes.

In addition to patient stories and testimonials that demonstrate successful outcomes, realistic expectations before and after the procedure are crucially addressed. Frequently asked questions and common concerns about thread lifts, such as pain

levels, duration of results, safety considerations, costs involved, and maintenance tips, are thoroughly addressed to equip readers with the knowledge they need to make an informed decision about their cosmetic journey.

CHAPTER ONE
THREAD LIFTS OVERVIEW
THREAD LIFT INTRODUCTION

Using dissolvable threads strategically placed beneath the skin to lift and support facial contours, a thread lift is a minimally invasive cosmetic procedure that rejuvenates sagging facial tissue. Unlike traditional facelifts, which involve surgery and longer recovery times, thread lifts use materials like PDO (polydioxanone) or PLLA (poly-L-lactic acid), which are biocompatible and stimulate collagen production. The threads are inserted using fine needles into the deeper layers of the skin, where they create a supportive structure that lifts sagging areas like the cheeks, jowls, brows, and neck.

Thread lifts are known for their natural-looking results and can be customized to suit each patient's unique facial anatomy and aesthetic goals. The procedure is performed under local anesthesia, making it relatively comfortable for the patient.

Once inserted, the threads provide an immediate lifting effect, and over time, they stimulate the body's natural collagen production, which further enhances skin elasticity and firmness. The threads gradually dissolve over several months, but the lifting effects can last up to 1-2 years depending on the type of threads used and individual skin characteristics.

ADVANTAGES OF LIFTING THREADS

With minimal downtime and faster recovery than traditional facelift surgery, thread lifts are an appealing non-surgical option for those seeking to address facial aging. Patients can return to normal activities a few days following the procedure. Thread lifts are also adaptable, as they can be used to lift different parts of the face, such as the cheeks, jawline, and brows, imparting a more youthful and lifted appearance without requiring extensive surgery.

A further advantage of thread lifts is that they produce results that are natural-looking. The threads not only raise sagging skin, but they also stimulate collagen production, which improves skin texture and firmness over time. For those who wish to improve their facial contours without the drastic changes that come with surgery, thread lifts are a good option because they are less invasive and involve less risk and complications than traditional facelifts.

A comprehensive evaluation by a medical professional is essential to ensure optimal results and safety. Patients considering thread lifts should speak with a qualified cosmetic surgeon or dermatologist to find out if they are good candidates for the procedure based on their skin condition, age, and aesthetic goals.

WHO IS ELIGIBLE FOR THREAD LIFTS?

Those with mild to moderate facial sagging who are seeking a non-surgical alternative to traditional facelift surgery can benefit most from thread lifts; ideal candidates will usually be in good general health and have reasonable expectations regarding the procedure's results.

Thread lifts can address issues like sagging cheeks, jowls, and brows, offering a subtle yet noticeable lifting effect that enhances facial contours and restores a more youthful appearance.

To ensure that the procedure is safe and appropriate for them, patients should discuss their medical history and any underlying health conditions with their cosmetic surgeon. Individuals who are pregnant or nursing, have certain medical conditions, or have unrealistic expectations about the procedure may not be ideal candidates for thread lifts. Candidates for thread lifts should also have good skin elasticity, as this contributes to the longevity of the results.

COMPREHENDING THE PROCESS

The thread lift procedure is carried out under local anesthesia in a clinical setting to ensure patient comfort. Using fine needles, the dermatologist or cosmetic surgeon strategically inserts dissolvable threads under the skin to lift and support sagging facial tissue, targeting areas like the brows, jawline, and cheeks to achieve a more youthful appearance.

Depending on the number of areas being treated and the complexity of the case, the procedure usually takes 30 minutes to an hour. The type and placement of threads used will depend on the patient's individual anatomy and aesthetic goals. Some threads are designed with barbs or cones that anchor into the skin to provide immediate lifting effects, while others stimulate collagen production over time for enhanced skin firmness and elasticity.

Most patients can resume normal activities and skincare routines shortly after the procedure, although strenuous exercise and exposure to direct sunlight should be avoided initially. The surgeon may gently massage the treated areas after the threads are inserted to ensure optimal placement and smooth results. Patients may experience mild swelling, bruising, or discomfort immediately after the procedure, but these side effects usually subside within a few days.

ANTICIPATIONS FOR THIS BOOK

In addition to covering important topics like selecting a qualified provider, getting ready for a thread lift, and managing expectations about the results, readers can expect to gain insights into how thread lifts work, who can benefit from them, and what to expect before, during, and after the procedure. This book aims to provide a comprehensive guide to understanding thread lifts, from their basic principles to detailed explanations of the procedure and its benefits.

This book aims to provide readers with the knowledge necessary to make educated decisions regarding facial rejuvenation procedures. Whether you're thinking about getting a thread lift for yourself or are just curious about non-surgical cosmetic options, it will be a useful resource for learning about the nuances of thread lifts and their role in contemporary aesthetic medicine.

CHAPTER TWO

THE FUNDAMENTALS OF THREAD LIFTS

THE MEANING AND BACKGROUND OF THREAD LIFTS

The idea for thread lifts began in Asia in the 1990s, when they were first used to treat facial sagging. The technique has evolved significantly, incorporating advanced thread materials and techniques to offer safer and more effective results. Thread lifts are a minimally invasive cosmetic procedure designed to lift and tighten sagging skin on the face, neck, and other areas. Using biocompatible threads, the procedure aims to stimulate collagen production, enhancing skin texture and firmness.

A stronger lifting effect and better skin anchorage are provided by barbed and cogged threads, which have improved the procedure's safety, effectiveness, and longevity. In the past, thread lifts were developed to meet the growing demand for less invasive alternatives to traditional facelifts. Early versions of the procedure used simple threads that were manually inserted into the skin, which frequently resulted in complications like thread breakage or visible marks.

In contrast to surgical facelifts, thread lifts are now hailed for their shorter recovery times and less downtime. The process usually entails using a fine needle or cannula to insert threads through tiny incisions, which are then tightened to lift and secure the skin in the desired position. The collagen that the body naturally produces surrounds the threads, strengthening the lift and improving skin elasticity. This makes thread lifts a desirable alternative for individuals seeking to rejuvenate their appearance without the invasiveness and drawn-out recovery associated with traditional surgery.

THREAD TYPES USED IN THREAD LIFTING

Thread lifts employ a variety of thread types, each intended to produce a distinct aesthetic result.

The most frequently utilized materials are PDO (Polydioxanone), PLLA (Poly-L-Lactic Acid), and PCL (Polycaprolactone). PDO threads are recognized for their safety and biocompatibility; they dissolve in six to twelve months while inducing collagen production; PLLA threads are longer-lasting, stimulating collagen growth for up to two years; therefore, they are perfect for more significant lifting effects; PCL threads, on the other hand, are the most recent materials available.

The threads in these materials are available in three different forms: smooth, barbed, and cogged. Barbed and cogged threads are equipped with small hooks or barbs that provide a firmer lift by anchoring the skin more securely.

These threads are strategically placed to lift sagging areas and create a contour that looks natural. The choice of thread is determined by the patient's skin condition, the desired lifting effect, and the specific areas to be treated. The practitioner customizes the technique for each patient.

A single thread may be inserted by some practitioners to address minor sagging, while multiple threads may be inserted by others for more extensive lifting. Tight control is exercised over the placement depth and tension of the threads to maximize benefits and minimize complications. More sophisticated techniques, like the "thread meshing" method, cross the threads in a grid pattern to enhance the lifting effect and promote collagen formation more uniformly. Customization guarantees that every patient receives a customized treatment plan, maximizing the benefits of the thread lift procedure.

COMPARISON TO OTHER PROCEDURES FOR FACIAL REJUVENATION

Though facelifts provide dramatic, long-lasting results, thread lifts are ideal for those seeking subtle enhancements with minimal downtime, making them suitable for younger individuals with early signs of aging. Compared to facelifts, fillers, and laser treatments, thread lifts are less invasive, requiring only small incisions or needle insertions; this significantly reduces the risk of complications, the need for general anesthesia, and the length of recovery time.

When compared to dermal fillers, which give the face volume, thread lifts are primarily used to lift and tighten sagging skin. Fillers can sometimes look unnatural if over-injected, but thread lifts stimulate collagen production, which offers a more gradual and natural improvement in skin texture and firmness. Laser treatments, while useful for tightening and resurfacing skin, do not have the same lifting effect as thread lifts. The combination of thread lifts and these treatments can improve overall skin quality and achieve comprehensive rejuvenation.

Among the non-surgical options available to patients are thread lifts, which offer instant lifting effects that get better with time as collagen grows around the threads; the procedure is adaptable, working on areas of the face and neck such as the jowls, nasolabial folds, and eyebrows; the short recovery period and minimal downtime make it a practical option for people with hectic schedules; and finally, patients can make decisions based on the pros and cons of thread lifts in comparison to other procedures.

RISKS AND SAFETY CONSIDERATIONS

Thread lifts are generally thought to be safe, but like any cosmetic procedure, there are possible risks involved. The most common side effects are mild bruising, swelling, and tenderness at the insertion sites; these usually go away in a few days. In rare instances, complications like infection, thread migration, or irregularities in the skin can happen. To reduce these risks, it is important to select a skilled and experienced practitioner who uses FDA-approved, high-quality threads and follows stringent hygiene and procedural standards.

To ensure they are a good candidate for the procedure, patients should discuss any pre-existing conditions and medical history with their practitioner. Risk factors for complications include diabetes, autoimmune disorders, and active skin infections. Smokers and people with poor skin quality may also have less satisfactory results. Complying with pre- and post-procedure instructions, such as avoiding strenuous activities and keeping the treated area clean, can significantly lower the risk of complications and improve the overall outcome of the thread lift procedure.

In addition, patients should be informed about the expected duration of their results and the possibility of future treatments to maintain the desired appearance. Follow-up appointments with the practitioner are crucial to monitor the progress and address any concerns promptly. Patients can benefit from thread lifts with confidence and peace of mind if they understand the safety aspects and take the necessary precautions.

DURATION AND ANTICIPATED OUTCOMES

Patients can usually expect noticeable improvements in skin tightness and contour from the day following the procedure.

The results are gradual, with optimal outcomes usually achieved within three to six months. This timeline allows the threads to fully integrate with the skin's tissue, enhancing the lifting and rejuvenating effects. Patients often experience a natural, youthful appearance without the telltale signs of surgery. Thread lifts offer immediate lifting effects, with the full benefits becoming more apparent as the collagen around the threads develops over the following weeks.

PDO threads typically last six to twelve months, while PLLA and PCL threads can maintain results for up to two or three years. One of the main benefits of thread lifts is the gradual absorption of the threads, which stimulates ongoing collagen production that continues to enhance skin texture and firmness even after the threads have dissolved. This sustained collagen stimulation is one of the main reasons for the longevity of the results, offering long-term skin rejuvenation beyond the initial lifting effect.

CHAPTER THREE

GETTING READY FOR THE THREAD LIFT

MEETING WITH A COSMETIC SURGEON FOR ADVICE

A consultation with a cosmetic surgeon is highly recommended before beginning a thread lift procedure. This first appointment has several functions, including a comprehensive evaluation of your medical history and present state of health; the surgeon will talk through your objectives and expectations regarding the thread lift, making sure they are within the scope of the procedure; you will also have the chance to ask questions regarding the procedure, possible risks, and anticipated results.

A personalized assessment is essential to ensure that the procedure is safe and effective for you. It also allows you to discuss any fears or concerns you may have about the procedure, which the surgeon can address and reassure you about.

The surgeon will examine the areas you wish to treat, assessing skin elasticity and overall facial structure to determine if you're a suitable candidate for a thread lift.

All things considered, the thread lift consultation with a cosmetic surgeon lays the groundwork for a positive experience. It gives you the knowledge you need to decide whether to proceed with the procedure and builds a trustworthy relationship with your healthcare provider for aftercare and support.

PRE-PROCEDURE INSTRUCTIONS AND LIMITATIONS

To maximize safety and outcomes, several guidelines and restrictions must be followed to prepare for a thread lift. Your cosmetic surgeon will go over these in detail during your consultation and in the days preceding your procedure. Generally, these guidelines include staying away from supplements and medications that may raise the risk of bleeding, such

as aspirin, ibuprofen, and certain herbal supplements.

It's important to closely adhere to these guidelines to minimize risks and ensure optimal conditions for the thread lift. In addition, you may be advised to stop smoking and limit alcohol consumption to promote better healing and reduce complications. Maintaining proper hydration and a healthy diet rich in vitamins and nutrients can also enhance your body's ability to recover post-procedure.

Comprehending and following these pre-procedure guidelines are essential stages in getting ready for a thread lift. They contribute to the creation of an atmosphere that is safe and conducive to the treatment, which in turn sets the stage for a more seamless recovery and better results.

COMPREHENDING THE PLAN OF TREATMENT

It's critical to comprehend your treatment plan in its entirety before having a thread lift. Your treatment plan will specify the precise areas of your body or face that will be treated, as determined by the cosmetic surgeon during your consultation. It is customized to your specific concerns and goals, guaranteeing that the threads are positioned strategically to produce the desired lifting and rejuvenating effects.

Understanding the mechanics of the procedure can ease your anxiety and help you visualize the expected results. Your cosmetic surgeon will go over the type of threads that will be used, whether they are absorbable or non-absorbable, and how they will be inserted beneath the skin to lift and support sagging tissues. The treatment plan also includes information about how long the procedure should take and what to expect right after.

You may go into the thread lift operation with confidence and reasonable expectations if you have a clear grasp of your treatment strategy. This clarity will improve your experience overall and help you achieve good aesthetic results.

BOTH MENTAL AND PHYSICAL READINESS

It takes more than just following instructions to ensure that you are mentally and physically ready for a thread lift procedure. To ensure that you are ready for the procedure as well as recovery, mentally prepare by visualizing the procedure and its results in a positive light, emphasizing the improvements you hope to achieve in terms of appearance. You can also discuss any concerns or worries you may have with your cosmetic surgeon, who can reassure you and allay them.

To prepare physically, you should maintain your general health and well-being. Getting enough sleep and rest before the procedure can help your body heal more quickly. Making sure you eat and drink right supports your immune system and helps repair damaged tissue. Some people find that deep breathing exercises or meditation help them relax before the procedure.

PUT OFF OR STEER CLEAR OF SUPPLEMENTS AND MEDICATIONS

Aspirin, ibuprofen, and some herbal supplements are examples of non-steroidal anti-inflammatory drugs (NSAIDs) that can thin the blood and cause increased bleeding during and after the procedure. Avoiding these medications and supplements in the days before your thread lift procedure can help prevent complications or interfere with the process.

To reduce the risk of excessive bleeding, bruising, or other side effects, your cosmetic surgeon will provide detailed instructions on which medications and supplements to avoid and for how long before the procedure. If you take prescription medications regularly, talk to your surgeon about whether any changes are needed before the procedure.

Following these recommendations shows that you are committed to getting the best results and guaranteeing a positive experience overall.

CHAPTER FOUR

PROCEDURE DAY ESSENTIALS

WHAT TAKES PLACE ON THE PROCEDURE DAY

When you show up at the clinic or facility on the day of your thread lift procedure, you should prepare by filling out any paperwork that needs to be completed. After that, you will be taken to a pre-procedure area where a healthcare provider will go over your medical history and answer any last-minute questions or concerns you may have. Finally, the practitioner will lead you to the procedure room where the thread lift will take place.

The area to be treated will be thoroughly cleaned to ensure sterility; depending on the type of thread lift chosen and the areas to be targeted, local anesthesia or numbing cream may be applied to minimize discomfort during the procedure. After you are in the procedure room, you will be asked to change into a gown or other appropriate attire and then positioned comfortably on the treatment table.

To achieve the desired rejuvenating effect, the actual procedure entails the insertion of threads under the skin using fine needles or cannulas; the practitioner will guide the threads into place, adjusting tension to achieve optimal results; once the procedure is finished, any excess threads will be trimmed, and the treated area will be inspected to ensure symmetry and the desired lift.

OPTIONS FOR ANESTHESIA AND PAIN CONTROL

The extent of the treatment area and your comfort level will determine which anesthetic is best for you. For thread lifts, local anesthesia is often used because it minimizes discomfort and allows you to remain awake and responsive during the procedure. Oral sedation is sometimes used in conjunction with local anesthesia to help you relax during the procedure.

The majority of patients find the discomfort tolerable, especially with the use of local anesthesia. Before beginning the procedure, the practitioner may apply a numbing cream to the skin to reduce the sensation of needle insertion. During the procedure, you may feel some pressure or mild discomfort as the threads are inserted and adjusted under the skin.

Your practitioner will provide specific instructions on post-procedure care and pain management to ensure your comfort and optimize healing. Some bruising, swelling, and minor discomforts at the thread insertion points are normal. After the procedure, any discomfort can usually be managed with over-the-counter pain relievers like acetaminophen.

OVERVIEW OF THE STEP-BY-STEP PROCEDURE

The thread lift procedure starts with marking the treatment areas and sterile drapes being applied to keep the area clean. After that, the practitioner numbs the area with local anesthesia or numbing cream to reduce discomfort. Then, using fine needles or cannulas, the threads are inserted under the skin.

The practitioner can lift and reposition sagging skin with a thread lift because the threads are equipped with tiny barbs or cones that grip the skin tissue. The threads are carefully guided into place, and tension is adjusted to achieve the desired lifting effect. Excess threads are trimmed, and the treated area is evaluated for symmetry and best outcomes.

Depending on the number of threads and treatment areas involved, the entire process usually takes one to two hours. You may have some mild discomfort and swelling immediately after the procedure, which is normal. After the threads are in place, the procedure is finished, and the treated area is cleaned and bandaged if necessary.

THE PROCESS'S DURATION

Depending on the intricacy of the treatment and the number of threads used, a thread lift procedure can take anywhere from one to two hours to complete. This can vary depending on the areas that need to be treated and the particular technique used by the practitioner. Thread lifts are usually minimally invasive procedures that can be finished in a single session at a clinic or medical spa.

To achieve the desired lifting and rejuvenating effect, the practitioner carefully places each thread during the procedure, which takes about an hour total and includes preparation, anesthetic administration, thread insertion, adjustment, and final inspection. Patients are encouraged to relax and stay as comfortable as possible throughout the procedure, which is intended to be efficient and effective in producing noticeable results.

Understanding the approximate duration of the procedure helps patients plan accordingly and feel more confident about undergoing a thread lift for facial rejuvenation or other aesthetic goals. Following the threads' insertion and adjustment, any excess threads are trimmed, and the treated area is cleaned and possibly bandaged. Your practitioner will provide specific instructions for post-procedure care to promote healing and optimize results.

INSTRUCTIONS FOR AFTERCARE STRAIGHT AFTER THE PROCEDURE

Following the post-procedural instructions given by your practitioner is crucial for promoting healing and achieving the best possible outcome following a thread lift procedure. You should expect some swelling, bruising, or mild discomfort around the thread insertion points, which can usually be managed with over-the-counter pain relievers such as acetaminophen.

Your practitioner may advise you to sleep with your head propped up on pillows to minimize swelling overnight, to avoid touching or moving the treated area excessively to allow the threads to settle in place, and to apply ice packs to the treated area intermittently for the first 24 hours to minimize swelling and discomfort.

Your practitioner may recommend gentle skincare routines and avoid saunas, hot tubs, and direct sun exposure until your skin has fully healed. For the first few days after the procedure, avoid heavy lifting, strenuous activities, and excessive facial movements that could strain the treated area.

You should make routine follow-up appointments with your practitioner to discuss any concerns and make sure the threads are settling correctly. If you carefully adhere to these aftercare instructions, you can promote a speedy healing process and get durable results from your thread lift procedure.

CHAPTER FIVE

HEALING AND FOLLOW-UP

THE FIRST PHASE OF RECOVERY

The initial recovery period following a thread lift procedure is critical to achieving the best possible outcome and minimizing discomfort. You should expect to have some mild swelling, bruising, and tenderness around the treated areas; this is normal and usually goes away in a few days. Your healthcare provider may prescribe over-the-counter pain relievers and ice packs applied gently to the treated areas to help manage discomfort; you should also avoid intense activities and excessive facial movements during this time to allow the threads to settle properly.

It's important to carefully follow your provider's post-procedure instructions to ensure a smooth recovery and the best possible outcome from your thread lift. During the first week, you should adhere to a gentle skincare routine recommended by your provider to promote healing and avoid disrupting the threads. This may involve using mild cleansers and avoiding harsh scrubs or exfoliants. Keeping your head elevated while sleeping can also help reduce swelling.

HANDLING PAIN AND SWELLING

Following a thread lift, there are a few doable strategies to help you get the most out of your recovery. First, you might experience some swelling and bruising around the treated areas; this is normal and usually goes away in a week or so. You can minimize swelling and ease any discomfort by applying cold compresses on and off during the first 24 to 48 hours. Your provider might also suggest gentle massages or lymphatic drainage techniques to improve circulation and lessen swelling.

As your body adjusts to the threads, you'll probably notice improvements in the contours and firmness of your skin over the next few weeks. It's important to avoid activities that could strain the facial muscles or increase blood flow to the treated areas, like vigorous exercise, sauna sessions, or excessive sun exposure. Taking prescribed or over-the-counter pain relievers as directed by your provider can also help manage any discomfort during the initial recovery phase.

ACTIVITIES AND RESTRICTIONS FOLLOWING PROCEDURE

After a thread lift, it is important to follow post-procedure instructions to minimize complications and achieve the best possible outcome. Your physician may recommend that you refrain from heavy lifting, vigorous exercise, and bending over for one to two weeks following the procedure because these activities can put a strain on your facial muscles and possibly loosen the threads before they have had time to settle in place.

A broad-spectrum sunscreen with SPF 30 or higher and avoiding prolonged exposure to sunlight are also necessary during the initial healing phase to protect your skin from UV rays, which can interfere with the healing process and cause pigmentation issues.

Your provider may also advise against using certain skincare products or treatments that could irritate your skin or disrupt the threads.

TIPS FOR LONG-TERM MAINTENANCE AND CARE

After the initial recovery period, you can gradually reintroduce regular skincare products and treatments recommended by your provider. These may include gentle cleansers, moisturizers, and serums designed to promote skin hydration and elasticity. Ultimately, maintaining the results of your thread lift over time requires having a comprehensive skincare routine and healthy lifestyle habits.

Regular follow-up appointments with your provider will allow them to assess your progress, address any concerns, and recommend additional treatments or adjustments as needed. Eating a balanced diet rich in antioxidants, vitamins, and minerals can also support skin health and collagen production, which contributes to the longevity of your thread lift results.

Protecting your skin from environmental stressors, such as pollution and UV radiation, by wearing sunscreen daily and using protective clothing can further enhance the effects of your thread lift.

RESCHEDULED VISITS AND EVALUATIONS

Following up with follow-up appointments and assessments is crucial for ensuring the best outcomes after a thread lift procedure. Your provider will schedule these appointments at predetermined intervals to assess how well the threads have settled and if any adjustments or additional treatments are needed. They may also take pictures, perform visual examinations, and talk with you about any concerns you may have regarding your skincare routine.

Your provider may recommend specific skincare products or treatments based on your skin type and concerns to enhance the longevity of your thread lift. By keeping these follow-up appointments and keeping lines of communication open with your provider, you can make sure that your thread lift results continue to live up to your expectations and that your skin stays healthy and rejuvenated. Additionally, these follow-up appointments offer you the chance to address any residual swelling or discomfort you may be experiencing and to receive personalized advice on maintaining your results.

CHAPTER SIX
ADVANTAGES OF LIFTING THREADS
BENEFITS OF SHORT-TERM AND LONG-TERM

For those seeking non-invasive facial rejuvenation, thread lifts provide both short-term and long-term benefits. Following the procedure, patients usually notice a slight lifting effect from the threads' immediate mechanical support, which can improve facial contours, particularly around the cheeks, jawline, and brows. As the threads stimulate collagen production, patients also notice longer-term improvements in skin elasticity and firmness, which further contribute to a more youthful appearance that improves in the months that follow the treatment.

These advantages make thread lifts an appealing choice for people looking to achieve noticeable facial rejuvenation with less risk and inconvenience than traditional surgery. Unlike surgical facelifts, thread lifts involve minimal downtime and recovery, allowing patients to resume daily activities almost immediately. Long-term benefits include sustained skin lifting and tightening effects as collagen continues to rebuild around the threads. This not only helps to maintain the initial results but also supports natural skin rejuvenation.

IMPACTS ON SKIN QUALITY AND FACIAL CONTOURING

By strategically placing absorbable threads beneath the skin, providers can lift and contour areas that have begun to droop, restoring a more youthful appearance. The threads create a scaffolding effect, lifting the skin and supporting tissues to redefine facial contours like the cheeks, jawline, and neck. Thread lifts have a significant impact on facial contouring and skin quality, addressing common signs of aging such as sagging skin and loss of facial volume.

Patients frequently report smoother, tighter skin that looks and feels rejuvenated. Unlike dermal fillers, which primarily focus on adding volume, thread lifts provide structural support, creating a natural and balanced facial contour that lasts. These effects not only improve aesthetic appearance but also boost self-confidence and satisfaction with one's facial appearance. Beyond lifting, thread lifts stimulate collagen production, which enhances skin quality over time. This leads to improvements in skin texture, elasticity, and overall firmness.

IMPACT ON THE MIND AND EMOTION

Thread lifts provide a non-surgical solution that restores a more youthful appearance, often leading to increased self-confidence and a more positive self-image. Patients report feeling more vibrant and refreshed after the procedure, which can positively influence their social interactions and overall well-being. The psychological and emotional impact of thread lifts can be profound for many individuals. Aging signs like sagging skin can impact self-esteem and confidence.

A thread lift can be a big deal for some patients as a turning point in their journey toward aging gracefully. The instantaneous improvement in skin quality and facial contours often translates to a renewed sense of youthful attractiveness, which can have a positive emotional impact on everything from professional relationships to personal relationships. Thread lifts effectively address visible signs of aging, giving people a sense of empowerment and self-confidence in their appearance.

POSSIBLE FINANCIAL SAVINGS WHEN COMPARED TO SURGERY

When compared to traditional surgical facelift procedures, thread lifts may be less expensive. The precise cost will vary based on the provider and the location, but overall, thread lifts are less expensive because they require less downtime and are less invasive.

Surgical facelifts can be very expensive because of the significant costs associated with anesthesia, hospital stays, and post-operative care. On the other hand, thread lifts are performed in-office under local anesthesia, which reduces associated costs.

Not only can patients return to normal activities within a few days, but the shorter recovery period associated with thread lifts also means fewer days away from work and reduced costs associated with post-operative care; this makes thread lifts not only a cost-effective option but also a convenient one for individuals with busy schedules. Thread lifts provide comparable aesthetic results without the high costs associated with surgery, making them an appealing alternative for patients on a budget seeking facial rejuvenation.

PATIENT CONTENTMENT AND TRIUMPHANT NARRATIVES

Success stories frequently highlight the natural-looking results achieved through thread lifts, which enhance facial contours while preserving the individual's unique features.

Patients appreciate the subtle yet noticeable improvements in skin tightness and smoothness, which contribute to a more youthful and refreshed look. Overall, patient satisfaction with thread lifts is high, with many people reporting positive outcomes and improved facial appearance.

Patients who have thread lifts report feeling rejuvenated and more confident in their appearance after the procedure; these testimonials highlight the procedure's ability to deliver satisfying results that meet patient expectations, making thread lifts a popular choice among those looking for non-surgical facial rejuvenation options. Many people who have thread lifts express satisfaction with the procedure's effectiveness in addressing their specific aging concerns. Success stories frequently highlight the minimal discomfort during the procedure and the relatively quick recovery period.

CHAPTER SEVEN

HAZARDS AND DIFFICULTIES

TYPICAL SIDE EFFECTS FOLLOWING THREAD LIFTS

The insertion points where the threads are placed under the skin may cause temporary swelling, bruising, and tenderness; these side effects usually go away in a few days to a week as the body gets used to the threads. Although thread lifts are generally safe, there are a few common side effects that beginners should be aware of. It's important to follow your healthcare provider's post-procedure care instructions to help minimize these effects.

In addition, mild discomfort or tightness in the treated area may occur initially but should go away as the threads integrate with the surrounding tissues; some patients may also experience slight puckering or dimpling of the skin where the threads are anchored, which usually smoothes out over time as the threads settle.

During the initial healing period, it is important to maintain good skin care practices and avoid applying pressure or making excessive facial movements on the treated area to promote optimal results.

An easier recovery process can be ensured by beginners knowing about these common side effects, which can help them prepare for what to expect post-thread lift. In rare instances, allergic reactions to the threads or local infections at the insertion sites may occur. These can usually be managed with appropriate medical treatment prescribed by your healthcare provider.

CONTROLLING AND REDUCING HAZARDS

A thorough consultation with a qualified healthcare provider is necessary before undergoing a thread lift procedure to manage and minimize the risks associated with the procedure. You should discuss your medical history, current medications, and expectations during the consultation to ensure that you are a suitable candidate for the treatment.

A proper assessment of your skin condition and realistic goals can help mitigate potential risks and complications.

A certified and experienced practitioner who uses FDA-approved threads and adheres to sterile techniques is essential. This lowers the risk of infection and guarantees that the threads are placed correctly for the best outcomes.

You can make an educated decision about whether to proceed with the treatment by being aware of the potential risks, which include asymmetry and thread migration.

Following the procedure, make sure you adhere to the post-care instructions that your healthcare provider has given you. This includes refraining from physically demanding activities, moving your face excessively, and staying out of direct sunlight for the prescribed amount of time. You should also schedule follow-up appointments as advised to monitor your recovery and address any concerns that may arise.

By being proactive, you can effectively manage and minimize the risks associated with thread lifts, ensuring a safer and more satisfying outcome.

POSSIBLE ISSUES AND STRATEGIES TO PREVENT THEM

Thread migration, in which the threads move from their original placement and cause asymmetry or visible irregularities in the treated area, is one potential complication that beginners should be aware of to make an informed decision. Fortunately, this can often be avoided by choosing an experienced practitioner who has expertise in thread lift procedures and uses advanced techniques to secure the threads properly.

An additional possible consequence is infection at the insertion sites, which can manifest as redness, swelling, or discharge. Strict sterile measures during the procedure and adherence to post-care instructions are essential to reduce this risk. Report any indications of infection to your healthcare provider as soon as possible so they can be evaluated and treated.

Furthermore, some people may have allergic reactions to the threads or the local anesthetic used in the procedure. Talk to your provider about any known allergies or sensitivities in advance to avoid negative reactions. Being aware of these possible side effects and taking precautions can help lower risks and improve the safety of having a thread lift procedure.

WHEN TO GET MEDICAL HELP

While mild swelling, bruising, and discomfort are common in the early post-procedure days, some symptoms may indicate complications that require medical evaluation. These include severe or increasing pain, excessive swelling that does not improve, persistent redness or warmth at the insertion sites, and fever. Knowing when to seek medical attention after a thread lift is crucial for ensuring proper recovery and addressing any unexpected issues promptly.

You must get in touch with your healthcare provider right away if you see any symptoms of infection, like pus or drainage coming from the insertion points. You should also seek medical advice for assessment and potential intervention if you notice any abrupt changes in the texture or appearance of your skin, like lumps, bumps, or asymmetry.

A safe and successful outcome from your thread lift can be ensured by being vigilant and proactive about your post-procedure symptoms. Follow-up appointments are typically scheduled to monitor your progress and address any concerns you may have during the recovery period.

Timely communication with your healthcare provider ensures that any issues are addressed promptly, minimizing the risk of complications and promoting optimal healing.

A LEGAL AND ETHICAL PERSPECTIVE

Before having a thread lift procedure, it is crucial to think about the ethical and legal implications of cosmetic procedures. You should also make sure that the clinic or facility where the procedure will be performed complies with health authorities' safety standards and regulations. Finally, make sure your healthcare provider is qualified, certified, and experienced in performing thread lifts to reduce risks and complications.

Understanding the possible risks, benefits, and alternatives of the procedure will help you make an informed decision based on realistic expectations and desired outcomes. Legal considerations include knowing your rights as a patient, including privacy and confidentiality of medical information, as well as recourse in the event of complications or unsatisfactory results. Have a thorough discussion about informed consent with your healthcare provider.

You can approach the procedure with confidence and peace of mind, knowing that your well-being and safety are prioritized, by addressing legal and ethical considerations before undergoing a thread lift. Ethical considerations include making sure that the procedure is performed with integrity, respecting your autonomy and dignity as a patient, and being transparent about pricing, including any additional fees for follow-up care or revision procedures.

CHAPTER EIGHT
SELECTING A CLINIC AND PROVIDER
LOOKING UP ELIGIBLE PROVIDERS

One of the most important things to do before beginning the process of getting a thread lift is to do your homework on qualified providers. Begin by making a list of possible clinics and practitioners who specialize in thread lifts.

Examine their credentials, including their medical licenses and certifications from reputable cosmetic surgery boards. These certifications validate their training and competence in performing thread lifts safely. Look for practitioners who have a lot of experience performing cosmetic procedures, especially thread lifts.

Then, look into their experience as a professional and reviews. Medical review websites, forums, and social media platforms are excellent sources of information about patient experiences.

Look for reviews that highlight the technical proficiency of the provider as well as their bedside manner and after-procedure care. If there are any negative reviews, take note of how the provider resolved them. You can also get referrals from family members or trusted friends who have had similar procedures.

Lastly, make an appointment for initial consultations with the providers you have narrowed down your options. This is an excellent time to evaluate the providers' communication style, responsiveness to your inquiries, and general patient care philosophy.

A quality provider will take the time to learn about your objectives, go over the procedure in detail, and address any worries you may have. By doing your homework and selecting a certified provider, you lay the groundwork for a positive thread lift experience.

EVALUATING CLINIC INFRASTRUCTURE AND ACCREDITATION

Assessing the clinic's accreditation and facilities in advance of a thread lift procedure is essential to guarantee a comfortable and safe experience. Start by looking at the facility's photos and description on their website; look for up-to-date, well-maintained facilities with the newest amenities and technology for outpatient procedures; clinics that place a high priority on cleanliness and organization enhance patient satisfaction and lower the likelihood of complications.

Another important thing to look for in a clinic is its accreditation. Find out if the clinic has been accredited by reputable medical associations or regulatory bodies. An accredited clinic follows strict guidelines for patient care, safety procedures, and procedural practices. This oversight helps guarantee that the facility meets or surpasses industry standards for emergency preparedness, hygiene, and equipment maintenance.

When you visit the clinic, observe the atmosphere and the professionalism of the staff. Knowledgeable, kind staff members who show consideration for patients' needs can make a big difference in how comfortable you feel about the whole experience. Examining the clinic's amenities and accreditation will boost your trust in the process as well as the medical staff that will be handling your care.

REVIEWS AND TESTIMONIALS FROM PATIENTS

When contemplating a thread lift procedure, it is crucial to learn about prior patients' experiences from reviews and testimonials. Start by looking for online forums where patients have posted their opinions about particular clinics and providers. Read through reviews that go into great detail about the patient's experience from consultation to recovery, emphasizing things like communication with the provider, comfort during the procedure, and satisfaction with the outcome.

Look for trends in reviews, taking note of any concerns or areas that need improvement that are brought up by several patients. Positive reviews that align with your expectations can give you confidence that you are selecting a reliable clinic and knowledgeable provider for your thread lift. On the other hand, take note of the clinic's response to negative reviews, as this shows that they are dedicated to patient satisfaction and ongoing improvement.

Ask the clinic for references or case studies of their prior thread lift procedures in addition to online reviews. Direct feedback from previous patients can provide insightful opinions on what to anticipate, including possible difficulties and post-procedure care advice. By carefully assessing patient reviews and testimonials, you obtain information that helps you make an educated choice and feel confident in your chosen clinic and provider.

WHAT TO ASK IN A CONSULTATION

To help you feel more clear-headed and confident about your decision to have a thread lift, prepare some questions for your consultation. Start by going over the specifics of the procedure, such as the kind of threads that will be used, the anticipated outcomes, and any risks or complications. By knowing these things, you can assess the provider's level of experience and their approach to customized treatment planning based on your particular aesthetic goals.

Find out about the provider's prior experience with thread lifts, including the number of procedures completed and success rates; this information will give you an idea of their skill level and track record in helping patients achieve their goals. You should also find out about the recovery process, including what to expect from the procedure, how long it will take to recover, and when you can go back to your regular activities.

Ask detailed questions during your consultation to make sure you are fully informed about the procedure, confident in your provider's abilities, and ready for every step of your thread lift journey. Discuss the cost of the procedure and what it includes, such as pre-operative consultations, anesthesia, and follow-up appointments. Clarify payment options, including whether the clinic accepts insurance or offers financing plans to accommodate your budget.

RECOGNIZING PRICES AND AVAILABLE PAYMENT METHODS

For financial planning and peace of mind, it is crucial to know pricing and payment options before moving forward with a thread lift procedure. To start, ask for a thorough cost breakdown during your consultation. This should include the surgeon's fee, facility fees, anesthesia fees, and any additional costs like pre-operative tests or medications. By knowing these costs upfront, you can budget appropriately and prevent financial surprises.

Discuss the viability of using health savings accounts (HSAs) or flexible spending accounts (FSAs) to cover eligible medical expenses related to the thread lift. Find out if the clinic accepts insurance for specific aspects of the procedure or if they provide documentation for reimbursement purposes. Find out about the clinic's available payment options. Some practices offer flexible financing plans or payment arrangements to help make elective procedures more affordable.

A skilled and experienced provider is essential for achieving satisfactory results and minimizing risks. By researching payment options and pricing beforehand, you can approach your thread lift procedure with confidence and concentrate on reaching your aesthetic goals. Compare pricing and payment policies among various providers to ensure you are receiving competitive pricing without compromising on quality or safety.

CHAPTER NINE

TREATMENTS OTHER THAN THREAD LIFTS

AN OVERVIEW OF FACE REJUVENATION WITHOUT SURGERY

To address common signs of aging such as fine lines, wrinkles, and loss of skin elasticity, non-surgical facial rejuvenation offers a variety of minimally invasive procedures that can be used to rejuvenate and revitalize the skin without the need for surgery. Some of the procedures that fall under this category are chemical peels, microdermabrasion, laser treatments, and thread lifts.

Particularly, dissolvable threads are carefully inserted into the skin to lift and support specific areas during a thread lift. This procedure stimulates collagen production, which further enhances skin firmness over time.

People who prefer minimal downtime over traditional surgical options frequently choose thread lifts because of their effectiveness in lifting and tightening sagging skin.

Selecting a non-surgical facial rejuvenation procedure requires an understanding of specific skin concerns and goals. Speaking with a qualified professional is essential to figuring out the best course of action based on skin type, desired results, and medical history. Non-surgical options are popular because they allow people to achieve natural-looking results without the risks of surgery.

COMPARING DERMAL FILLERS AND BOTOX

Understanding the distinctions between thread lifts, Botox, and dermal fillers is crucial when considering non-surgical options for facial rejuvenation. Botox, a neurotoxin, smoothes targeted areas by blocking nerve signals that cause muscle contractions, giving the appearance of smoother, younger-looking skin for several months. It temporarily paralyzes facial muscles to reduce the appearance of dynamic wrinkles like crow's feet and forehead lines.

On the other hand, dermal fillers, which are often used to plump lips, enhance cheekbones, and fill deep lines, use hyaluronic acid or other biocompatible substances to add volume and structure to areas affected by static wrinkles or loss of facial volume. Depending on the type of filler used, the results can be seen right away and last for several months to over a year.

Unlike fillers and Botox, which require repeated treatments to maintain results, thread lifts can offer longer-lasting effects with proper care and maintenance, making them appealing to those looking for a semi-permanent solution to facial aging. Unlike fillers and Botox, which physically lift and realign sagging skin and tissues, thread lifts provide a subtle but noticeable lift that improves over time as collagen production is stimulated.

MODIFICATIONS TO LIFESTYLE FOR SKIN HEALTH

Beyond cosmetic procedures, achieving and maintaining optimal skin health involves implementing healthy lifestyle practices that support skin vitality from the inside out. For example, drinking plenty of water every day is crucial to maintaining skin elasticity, and a balanced diet rich in vitamins, antioxidants, and essential fatty acids supports the production of collagen and helps combat oxidative stress, which can accelerate the aging process of the skin.

Preventing sunburns, premature aging, and skin cancers can be achieved by wearing hats, finding shade during peak sun hours, and maintaining a consistent skincare routine that is customized to the specific needs of each person. This routine should include cleansing, exfoliating, moisturizing, and using targeted treatments such as masks or serums to promote skin health and maximize the benefits of professional treatments.

Reducing cortisol levels, which can lead to collagen degradation and skin inflammation, is one way that stress management practices like yoga, meditation, or deep breathing help maintain healthy skin. Getting enough sleep is another important way to help maintain healthy skin because it gives the skin time to repair and regenerate which minimizes the appearance of fatigue and fine lines and leaves the complexion looking more rested.

COMBINATION THERAPIES TO IMPROVE OUTCOMES

For those seeking a more complete facelift, combining various non-surgical procedures can yield better and more personalized outcomes. This technique, which is frequently customized by trained professionals, targets several issues at once, including wrinkles, volume loss, and skin laxity, for a cohesive final appearance. For example, combining dermal fillers for volume restoration and Botox for dynamic wrinkles can produce a youthful, well-proportioned appearance.

Combining thread lifts into a combination treatment plan gives a lifting and firming aspect that enhances the effects of other procedures. Practitioners can maximize results while minimizing recovery times and downtime by layering treatments strategically according to each patient's needs. This is especially advantageous for patients with complex aging concerns or those seeking noticeable but natural-looking improvements in facial aesthetics.

A qualified aesthetic provider can offer recommendations for the best treatment combinations based on skin type, desired outcomes, and budget, ensuring a customized approach that maximizes patient satisfaction and results. Consulting with a qualified aesthetic provider is essential for creating a personalized treatment plan that addresses specific goals and concerns comprehensively.

CUSTOMIZING THERAPY PROGRAMS

Customization of non-surgical facial rejuvenation treatments entails evaluating each patient's distinct skin traits, concerns, and intended results to develop a customized plan. This personalization guarantees that treatments effectively target particular signs of aging while taking into account variables like skin type, lifestyle, and medical history. The first step in identifying the best procedures and techniques is a comprehensive consultation with a qualified professional.

To make the best treatment recommendations, the practitioner assesses the patient's skin texture, elasticity, volume loss, and wrinkle severity during the consultation. Aside from the patient's expectations and lifestyle, other considerations that impact the treatment plan include the patient's budget and desired downtime. Practitioners who involve their patients in the decision-making process build trust and collaboration, which improves treatment outcomes and patient satisfaction.

Frequent follow-up appointments and skincare recommendations further support long-term maintenance and enhancement of results, promoting ongoing skin health and vitality. Personalized treatment plans may involve a series of sessions spaced over time to achieve gradual improvements and allow for skin adaptation between treatments. This phased approach also allows for adjustments based on how the skin responds to initial treatments, ensuring optimal results while minimizing potential risks or complications.

CHAPTER TEN

REASONABLE ANTICIPATIONS AND PATIENT NARRATIVES

BEFORE TREATMENT, ESTABLISH REASONABLE EXPECTATIONS

To ensure a positive experience and outcome following a thread lift procedure, it is important to have realistic expectations about what the procedure can realistically achieve. Unlike invasive surgeries, thread lifts offer subtle improvements by lifting sagging skin and promoting collagen production. To ensure you have a clear understanding of what to expect, it is important to consult with a qualified practitioner who can assess your skin's condition and discuss achievable results based on your unique needs. During the consultation, factors such as skin elasticity, age, and desired outcomes will be taken into account.

It's also important to be realistic about the degree of improvement and the duration of results; most thread lifts offer immediate lifting effects with ongoing improvements in skin texture and firmness over several months. By going over these details with your practitioner and coming into the procedure with realistic expectations, you can approach the procedure with confidence and a clear understanding of its benefits. Thread lift limitations: Although they can offer noticeable rejuvenation, they are not a substitute for more invasive procedures like facelifts.

ACCOUNTS OF TRIUMPHANT THREAD LIFT RESULTS

Reading accounts of positive thread lift results can be a great way for people to think about getting one. Many patients talk about how they were able to achieve natural-looking results with little downtime. These accounts show how the thread lifts lifted and tightened their facial contours, which helped with mild to moderate sagging in the brows, cheeks, or jowls. Successful results also highlight how subtle and natural the enhancement is from thread lifts, which appeals to people looking for rejuvenation without going overboard.

The thread lift's ability to lift sagging skin and stimulate collagen production has been attributed by patients to feeling more youthful and confident after the procedure. Seeing before-and-after photos of people with similar concerns can further illustrate the potential benefits of a thread lift. These first-hand accounts and visual evidence can help prospective patients visualize their potential results and feel more informed about what to expect from the procedure.

IMAGES AND TESTIMONIALS FROM BEFORE AND AFTER

The effectiveness of thread lifts is largely demonstrated by before and after photos, patient testimonials, and real-world transformations that highlight how the procedure can improve skin laxity and enhance facial contours. Before photos usually highlight initial concerns, such as sagging skin or lost definition in the jawline or cheeks, while after photos show the immediate lifting effects and gradual improvements in skin tone and texture after the procedure.

Viewing these photos and reading patient testimonials can give prospective patients a realistic preview of what the procedure can achieve and help them make an informed decision about having a thread lift. Patients' testimonials often accompany these photos, sharing their journey from initial consultation to post-procedure recovery. They highlight their motivations for choosing a thread lift, their experience during the treatment, and the outcomes they achieved. Many testimonials emphasize the natural-looking results and the boost in self-esteem they gained from their enhanced appearance.

EFFECTS OF AESTHETIC TREATMENTS ON THE MIND

Aesthetic treatments, such as thread lifts, have a psychological impact that goes beyond physical changes to include emotional and mental well-being. A lot of people seek these procedures to deal with insecurities or signs of aging that negatively impact their self-confidence. Aesthetic treatments, such as thread lifts, can help patients have a positive outlook on appearance and a positive self-image.

Patients who have successful treatments report feeling more empowered and confident, which can improve social interactions and career opportunities.

Patients and practitioners can work together to achieve desired aesthetic improvements while supporting emotional well-being by fostering open communication and setting achievable goals. Practitioners play a significant role in addressing patient concerns and providing reassurance throughout the treatment process.

However, it's important to recognize that psychological responses and expectations vary among individuals. Managing expectations and understanding realistic outcomes are crucial to avoid disappointment and ensure satisfaction with the results.

ADVICE ON HANDLING EXPECTATIONS AFTER SURGERY

Immediately following treatment, some swelling and bruising are normal, but these usually go away within a few days to a week. Patients are advised to follow post-procedure care instructions provided by their practitioner, which may include avoiding strenuous activities and applying cold compresses to reduce swelling. Managing expectations post-thread lift procedure involves understanding the recovery process and realistic timelines for seeing final results.

People can maximize the benefits of their thread lift and experience long-lasting rejuvenation by being informed and patient throughout the healing process. It's important to keep in mind that thread lifts offer gradual improvements over several months as collagen production increases and skin continues to tighten.

Patience is key during this period, and maintaining realistic expectations about the pace of results can help manage satisfaction. Regular follow-up appointments with your practitioner allow for monitoring progress and addressing any concerns that may arise.

CHAPTER ELEVEN

FREQUENTLY ASKED QUESTIONS

DO THREAD LIFTS CAUSE PAIN?

Because they are less invasive than traditional surgical facelifts, thread lifts are generally thought to be minimally painful procedures. Local anesthesia is usually used to ensure minimal discomfort during the procedure, and the fine threads that are used are intended to be inserted smoothly under the skin to lift and support tissues. Some patients may feel a slight tugging sensation during the procedure, but this is usually temporary and well-tolerated.

Overall, most people find thread lifts to be a manageable and relatively comfortable procedure with little downtime. Mild soreness or bruising may occur post-procedure, which can be managed with over-the-counter pain relievers and ice packs. It's important to follow post-operative care instructions provided by your healthcare provider to minimize any discomfort and ensure optimal healing.

WHAT IS THE DURATION OF RESULTS?

Results from a thread lift can last anywhere from one to three years, depending on several factors such as the type of threads used and the unique characteristics of each patient's skin.

Threads made of materials such as PDO (polydioxanone) are gradually absorbed by the body, which stimulates collagen production and improves skin texture and firmness over time.

How long the effects of a thread lift procedure last can depend on several factors, including lifestyle choices, skin care regimen, and the aging process. Some people choose to have touch-up procedures or additional threads to maintain or enhance results, while others choose to follow recommended skin care practices and lead a healthy lifestyle.

ARE ALL USERS SAFE WHEN USING THREAD LIFTS?

For healthy people looking to improve mild to moderate signs of facial aging, thread lifts are generally safe. But, you should speak with a qualified healthcare provider to find out if you're a good candidate for the procedure, as some medical conditions or skin conditions may prevent you from having a thread lift.

Candidates who have unreasonably high expectations for the procedure's results are pregnant or nursing, have an active skin infection, or are otherwise unfit candidates may not be considered.

Your healthcare provider will thoroughly review your medical history and evaluate your skin condition to determine whether the thread lift procedure will be safe and effective for you.

WHAT ARE THE ASSOCIATED COSTS?

A thread lift procedure can cost anywhere from a few hundred to several thousand dollars per session, depending on several factors including the clinic's location, the experience level of the healthcare provider, the number of threads used, and the complexity of the treated area.

During your initial consultation, you must discuss pricing with your healthcare provider. They can offer you a detailed breakdown of costs, including any additional fees for anesthesia, post-procedure care, and follow-up appointments. A procedure may be more affordable if the clinic offers financing options or packages for multiple sessions.

HOW TO SUSTAIN OUTCOMES OVER TIME

To preserve the results of a thread lift procedure, you should follow a regular skin care regimen and adopt healthy lifestyle practices. These include using sunscreen daily, drinking plenty of water, abstaining from tobacco use, and using skincare products and moisturizers that have been prescribed by your physician to nourish and protect your skin.

Aside from that, making follow-up appointments as directed by your physician enables them to evaluate your progress and suggest any touch-up procedures or adjustments that may be necessary. Some patients may find that additional treatments, like dermal fillers or laser skin rejuvenation, help to prolong and improve the results of their thread lift.

You may extend the benefits of a thread lift operation and keep your skin looking young and renewed for a longer time by caring for your skin proactively and by following your doctor's advice.

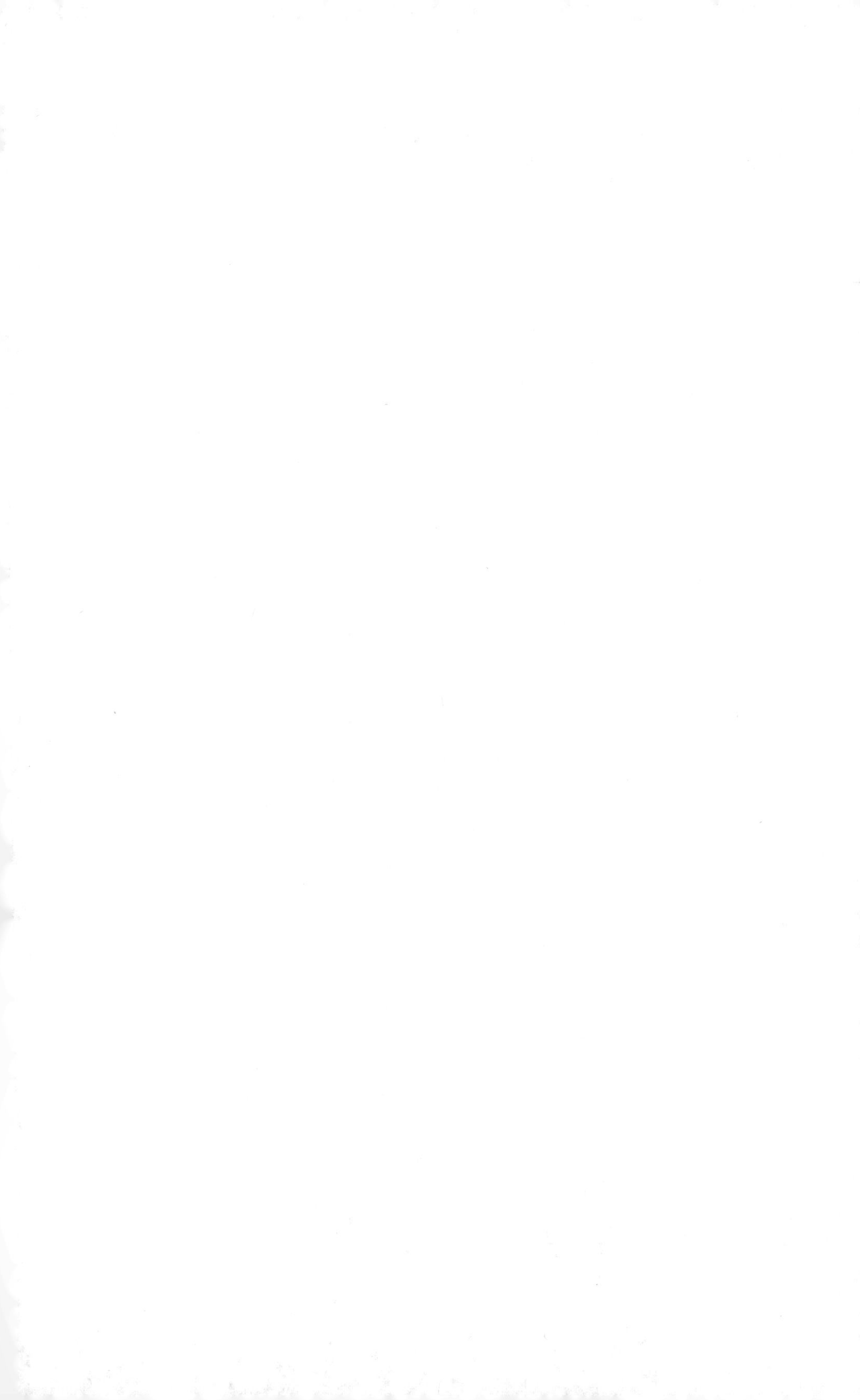

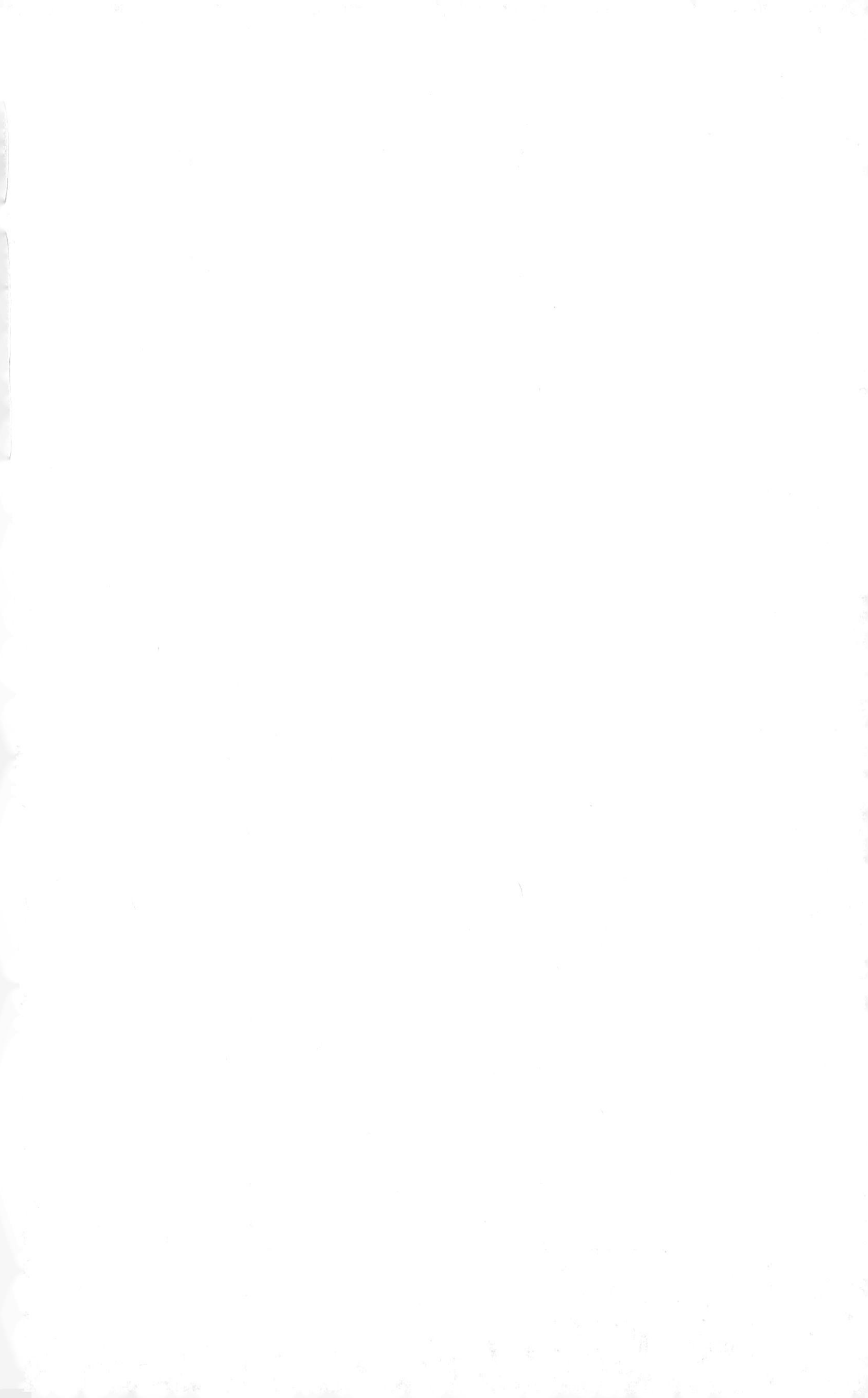